THE BRAIN
THAT CHANGES EVERYTHING

Get Smarter ● Think Faster ● Live Better

The 59 Minute Guide to Accelerating Your Brain

Shaahin Cheyene

www.excelerol.com

A Shaahin Cheyene Paperback

First published in the USA in 2012 by Accelerated Intelligence Inc.

Copyright © 2012 Shaahin Cheyene

The right of Shaahin Cheyene to be identified as the author of this work has been asserted in accordance with the Copyright, Designs & Patents Act 1988.

All rights reserved. No part of this publication may be reproduced, stored in a retrieval system, or transmitted, in any form or by any means, internet, electronic, mechanical, photocopying, recording or otherwise, without the prior permission of the owner.

ISBN: 146804009X

ISBN-13: 978-1468040098

Typeset in Garamond & Myriad Pro

Liability

No responsibility or liability is assumed or accepted by the author for any claimed financial losses and/or damages sustained to persons from the use of the information in this publication, personal or otherwise, either directly or indirectly. While every effort has been made to ensure reliability and accuracy of the information within, all liability, negligence or otherwise, from any use, misuse or abuse of the operation of any methods, strategies, instructions or ideas contained in the material herein, is the sole responsibility of the reader. By reading past this point you are accepting these terms and conditions.

Medical Disclaimer

This book is a reference manual intended to promote informed choices of the reader. I am not a doctor or a medical professional. This book does not endorse a particular product or type of treatment. This book is intended for educational purposes only. This book should not be used as a manual for self-diagnosis. This book and the advice within are not intended to treat, cure, prevent or diagnose any disease. Always consult a health care professional when faced with any persistent symptoms, acute pain, or disability. Neither the author nor publisher assumes responsibility for the misuse of any and all information contained in this book.

CONTENTS

FOREWORD 7
INTRODUCTION 11
    Foundations of Intelligent Decisions 12
    The Power of Focus 12
    Heisenberg Uncertainty Principle 14
    How to Use This Book 14
ACCELERATED DEVELOPMENT 16
NEUROPHYSIOLOGY 18
    Evolving Brains 18
    Elasticity and Plasticity 19
    Neural Networks 20
    Expanding Your Neural Network 20
    Learning Boosts Brain Power 21
    Cortisol 22
THE THREE KEYS 23
    1. Memory 23
    2. Focus, Concentration & Alertness 23
    3. Your Processing Speed 24
FOUR TIER APPROACH 25
    1. Diet & Nutrition 25
    2. Exercise 25
    3. Supplements 26
    4. Mental Exercise 26

1. NUTRITION 27
    The Energy of Thought and Memory 28
    Protein 29
    Top Ten Protein Rich Foods 29
    Top 10 Vegetarian Protein Rich Foods 30
    Omega 3 Fatty Acids 31
    High Protein & Slow Carbs 31
    Top 10 Brain Foods 33
    10 Foods to Throw Out 34
    Eating For Intelligence 35
2. EXERCISE 39
    Top Ten "RESTING TO RAPID" Exercises 40
    Move It or Lose It 41
    Walking 42
    Running 43
    Aerobic Exercise 44
    Exercise Tips 45
3. BRAIN BOOSTERS 47
    Nootropics / Neuroprotectives 51
    Adaptogens 53
    Stimulants 54
4. MENTAL EXERCISE 58
    A Simple Brain Exercise 58
    Top 10 Brain Exercises 59
    Travel 60
    Neurobic Exercises 60

Taking Care of Your Brain 64
30 SECOND OVERVIEW 69
FURTHER READING 70
EXCELEROL 72
NEURODRIN 74
ACCELERATED INTELLIGENCE DIGITAL PILL
    DISPENSER 75
NEURODRIN INHALER 76
ABOUT THE AUTHOR 77

FOREWORD

Reading a book by someone who has really lived this stuff is far more interesting than the dry science to which we are often subjected. Before we begin our journey, I'd like to share my story with you. I believe this will give you a clear picture of me and my personal path. I am devoted to life expansion, cognitive enhancement, personal achievement, and healing. It will also allow you to see what motivated me to begin my journey in the first place. It is my hope that you will find the inspiration to begin improving your own brain.

For at least five generations, both of my grandfathers (from Iran) were master herbalists, dedicated to life extension and naturopathic medicine. We moved to the States during the Iranian Revolution.

I left home when I was fifteen. Before my sixteenth birthday, I met a mysterious shaman who changed my life. I spent nearly a year apprenticing with this man and learning everything ranging from life lessons to herbal medicine. Although I have been taking herbs since I was a child, it is only since my apprenticeship at age sixteen that I began to create and use my own formulations.

During my apprenticeship with this amazing man, I was taught about the secrets of good nutrition, exercise, and supplementation. I learned how to expand my brain naturally. It has paid off.

In the early 1990's, shortly after my apprenticeship with little or no money and no formal education, I invented an herbal supplement that would prove to be a game changer. I solicited the help of scientists, herbalists, and naturopaths like the great naturopathic doctor, Andrew Weil, M.D., who graciously entertained my long-winded phone calls, probing for knowledge in the field.

The product became known as Ecstacy (intentionally misspelled) or Herbal Ecstacy. It was my own version of real Ecstasy. However, mine was made strictly from herbs. It completely legal, and, being all-natural, had none of the pharmaceutical Ecstasy's side effects.

It sounds incredible, but I started with only a borrowed $1,000. In less than a month I turned it into $100,000. With that, I was able to perfect the product. I reduced it to five tiny tablets emblazoned with a butterfly on one side and an "e" on the other. I printed slick marketing materials – brochures and posters – and produced electric rave packaging. The crowds ate it up – literally!

Within a year, we were reported to have made over $300 million dollars in sales. I was a teenage millionaire! We opened offices in five countries. The product was unavoidably pervasive no matter where you looked. At the time, there was nothing else like it on the market. We had created the world's first natural, smart pill.

All this was happening during the internet boom. Amongst many other uses, we noticed that programmers, internet entrepreneurs and laymen alike were taking the pills to boost their cognitive performance. We had sparked the "smart pill" revolution.

Shortly thereafter, I expanded the Herbal Ecstacy brand, adding over 200 different products, including a highly-successful herbal cigarette line that was once the object of a bidding war between two large tobacco companies. I left the Ecstacy business and took a year off. As a by-product of my research, I then developed a revolutionary new drug delivery technology called the "Vapir Vaporizer."

I accomplished many far-reaching goals. I published a successful magazine (with over 100,000 issues in circulation), and appeared on many television shows including "Prime Time" with Sam Donaldson, "The Montel Williams Show" and "Seattle's Town Hall. I was photographed by David LaChapelle and enjoyed being on the cover of *Newsweek* three times. Additionally, my products and I were the subjects of countless other cover stories for hundreds of other magazines and newspapers. I was interviewed on several major television and radio networks including: the BBC, NBC, ABC, CNN, CNBC, and MTV.

I also traveled extensively, researching native cultures and their medicines. I imported artifacts and other strange objects from India and Thailand. I opened an Ecstacy retail store franchise with hundreds of stores. I discovered a supply for a strange, ancient, Mexican plant medicine and was the first to import it on a mass scale to the United States. I experimented with every major (and minor) plant medicine from around the world and conducted interviews and extensive research on cognitive enhancement technologies worldwide. I then invented modern digital vaporization and about 200 other products. Many were hugely successful and paradigm shifting.

Neurodegenerative disease is something that affects us all. As we get older, our brains degrade and we lose the function and structure of our neurons. In the best case, this is occasional brain fog that we all experience from time to time. With the technology now available to us, this brain degradation can be prevented and, in some cases, reversed. I have spotted many trends and spent over fifteen years studying different scientists, healers, and shamans all over the world.

For the past five years, I have been working on solutions to the challenges of aging and of brain function deterioration. In recent months, my company has had a few major breakthroughs. My quest is not entirely altruistic. As I am getting older myself, I see a real need to stop the potential damages from neurodegenerative diseases. For this reason, I have dedicated the next several years to developing technologies and products to improve brain function, slow aging, accelerate intelligence, and halt neurodegenerative disease.

This all came together in this book. Everything I have learned about cognitive enhancement and through herbalism, chemistry, physiology, psychology, and the power of the mind has been distilled into this guide to boosting your cognitive ability. It's time we shift the paradigm. It's time we get better and smarter.

INTRODUCTION

This is the ultimate guide to discovering your superhuman brain. If you take just an hour out of your busy schedule to read this book, you'll be well on your way to improving your brainpower. I've condensed all the fastest, most powerful techniques into one, easy-to-follow guide.

The book is based on a simple concept. Contrary to what was believed in the past, neurobiology has proven, in recent years, that our brains are plastic and changeable. We can alter not only our brain chemistry, but the way that our brains work. We can achieve and maintain what I like to call a "super genius state" every day of our lives. Changing our brains can change everything.

Placebos are drugs without any active ingredients. They are used in testing new medicines, to show the difference between a patient who takes the active ingredient and a patient who takes nothing but is unaware of this. The power of our minds is truly limitless. Doctors and scientists have found the effectiveness of placebos is growing with each day. The amazing thing is that many people's health actually improves when they take a placebo. Why?

Could it be because, when you pay attention to any area of your life, it improves? Do you believe that the brain is so powerful that it can affect the body in amazing ways? Do people who take a placebo find benefits because their mind truly believes they will get better, and because the placebo has focused their mind on the problem?

Becoming a super genius is all about focusing on your brain, believing that it is improving, and taking concerted action to improve your most valuable asset.

Foundations of Intelligent Decisions

The medical community and drug manufacturers have been rocked many times by the amazing effect of placebos. The first clue came from Fabrizio Benedetti at the University of Turin. He documented trial after trial where expensive, new pharmaceuticals got trounced by patients taking placebos.

Similar studies were done by institutions like Harvard Medical School. Harvard investigated over a thousand patients. From theirs and other studies, it has become evident that placebos have a potentially unlimited degree of therapeutic effectiveness.

The Power of Focus

After years of consulting with hundreds of people on the best course of naturopathic and herbal remedy for their conditions, I noticed an unusual thing. I would often recommend a synergistic course of treatment that involved three areas: nutrition, exercise, and supplementation. Often, people disregarded the advice and chose only one of the areas on which to focus. I knew that, often, they could have quickly and drastically improved their conditions if they followed the three-part plans I set for them. However, I began to notice that they, in fact, were experiencing a substantial degree of improvement after deciding to take action. This was despite the fact that they often did not move past the initial decision stage.

What was even stranger is that a fifty-eight-year-old New York lawyer whom we will call Joe, whom I had consulted, had suffered from a severe memory condition. Joe started to go into remission almost instantaneously after our sessions together. I had put together a meticulously mapped out plan for Joe. I knew from his personality that he was not following the entire three-part plan. So, I was curious to see just how much of my plan he was actually following.

I met with Joe at his home some weeks later. After searching his refrigerator and reviewing his journal with him, I noticed that he had not followed the plan at all. In fact, what he had done was to create his own "hybrid" of the plan I had set for him. He vaguely followed it when he felt like it. His version of my carefully planned scheme was the medical equivalent of eating a banana while being suspended upside down in a vat of butter. But that is neither here nor there. The fact remained that he experienced a substantial improvement in his condition, even though he did not do most of the program that I recommended.

I began to investigate several other clients and noticed that many had gone through a similar pattern and achieved similar results. This brought me to a shocking realization. The only real variable in the lives of these people was that they decided to pay attention to an area of their life that they had previously been ignoring.

It brought me to the stark realization that when you give positive attention to any area of your life, then that area grows and improves. Any attention to an area has a more dramatic impact than no attention. You may not instantly be able to cure every condition, but you surely can improve a condition simply by giving attention to that area. The decision to take action is a quantifiable step in any plan.

Heisenberg Uncertainty Principle

I later learned that this may be explained by the Heisenberg Uncertainty Principle. In 1927, a German scientist named Werner Heisenberg proved that sub-atomic particles behave differently when observed. The process of observing appears to influence what is being observed.

What this means to you and me, is that as we focus on any area of our lives, the act of appreciation and measurement of your progress may very well be creating the very reality it is measuring. The more you focus, the more solid the reality you create. Physics thus explains theoretically what I had experienced directly.

How to Use This Book

Any philosophy worth taking on can be learned quickly. After all, it does me no good if you age by the time you read this. The brain retains the most information in the first and last five minutes of any session. This book was designed to be read in a total of two fifty-nine-minute sessions. I recommend five-minute increments with a one- minute break in between.

I've kept the heavy science to a minimum and focused on practical ways to improve your mind power. This is a pragmatic guide based on real things you can do right now to improve your brain. Training your brain needn't be a tough, intensive process. This book will make your journey fun. Above all, I want to get you pumped and excited about how powerful your new brain could be. So flip through, and learn some simple ways to discover your super genius brain.

ACCELERATED DEVELOPMENT

The whole human race is changing. We are living longer, and aging more slowly. The whole demographic of our world is being altered. People like Jeanne Louise Calment, the hundred-and-twenty-two-year-old from Arles in France, have pushed the limits of longevity. She was the longest living person in recorded history. She certainly did not look her age. When you think that only a few generations ago, a lifetime usually ended at forty, this is remarkable.

Or, consider Jack LaLanne, the "Godfather of Fitness", who at age fifty-four, beat a twenty-one-year-old Arnold Schwarzenegger in an informal bodybuilding contest. He showed millions of fitness fans just how far he could push the envelope with the body. At seventy, he was handcuffed, shackled, and roped to seventy rowboats, which he then towed one mile, swimming in high winds and dangerous currents.

At the other end of the spectrum we have seen equally amazing advances in regeneration of the brain. Stroke victims, people with severe disabilities, and even blindness have all seen huge improvements using cutting edge techniques.

Today forty is the new thirty, and fifty is the new forty. The rate at which we age and deteriorate may be slowing exponentially. Looking and feeling amazing at an age most people used to think of as retirement age has become a modern phenomenon. The old assumptions about what is possible are being eroded. Total life expectancy is increasing with every generation.

At the same time, we are seeing youngsters entering university at age twelve, and an increasing number of child prodigies. At both ends of the spectrum, the human race is advancing, fast. This goes to show how much hidden potential we have inside us. The key is learning how to unlock this potential and put it to use in our daily lives.

What we are seeing are the results of improved diet, healthcare, and new mental attitudes which are literally accelerating the development of the human race. These same factors can be brought to bear directly on your own mind and body, and you can expect similarly spectacular results.

NEUROPHYSIOLOGY

Although neurophysiology is a large word and sounds complex, its meaning is simple. Basically, neurophysiology is the study of the function of our brain. This includes all electric and chemical reactions that allow us to function in our day-to-day lives.

Contrary to more antiquated scientific theories, the brain isn't set in its permanent state at birth. In fact, the brain is a living organism that develops and grows throughout our lifetime. This process is known as "neuro-plasticity."

The brain is an adaptable organ, capable of handling the most difficult tasks under the least opportune conditions. For example, one famous experiment showed that people with visual challenges when provided with certain sensory inputs via vibrations or touch, could recognize visual descriptions. Now, with the right knowledge and technology anyone can successfully deal with many cognitive problems or deficiencies, as well as expand a normal and healthy brain. Anything is possible.

Our old assumptions about the brain being fixed and non-bending were way off the mark.

Evolving Brains

The progressive development of the human brain has been nothing short of extraordinary. Imagine — if you will — pre-historic earth. The primitive life forms that inhabited our oceans had neither nerve cells, nor a brain that permitted them to move. In fact, sponges and other primitive beings merely waited for their food to float past.

However, through time, a new form of life came into existence. Beings developed nerve cells and, later, full brains that could command movement. Life forms, such as jellyfish and sea anemones that advanced past the stage of simple organisms, developed simple nervous systems and were finally able to locate their food and hunt it. Accordingly, this process implemented both a phenomenal change and a tremendous evolutionary advantage.

Consequently, the brain came into existence, and since then, it's been the major deciding factor between animals surviving and those that become extinct. Indeed, we as human beings, as frail as we are, have not only managed to forgo extinction, we've managed to rise to the most powerful form of life on the planet. Why? Many believe it is because of our extraordinary brain potential.

Elasticity and Plasticity

Your brain is both elastic and plastic. Elasticity refers to the ability of something to return to its original shape after being stretched. For example, your muscles easily snap back to their starting position during exercise. The elastic properties of our brains give us a flexible approach to thinking.

Plastic means something which can be molded. Just like clay, you can mold your brain into new, more powerful shapes by training and conditioning it. The plastic properties of our brains give us a programmable approach to our thinking.

Neural Networks

Your neural networks, or neural connection pathways, began to develop while you were in the womb. In fact, you create 15,000,000 neural connections every hour, to build a network of 100,000,000,000 neurons. This network used to be thought of as fixed, reaching a peak during our teenage years. Now, we know that we can expand and forge new connections in our neural network throughout our lives. Even damaged brains can be developed to rebuild neural connections. The more connections, and the more complex the matrix, the greater your intelligence.

Expanding Your Neural Network

The brain feeds on novel experiences. Seek them out, and you feed your super genius brain. Each time that you experience something that's new to you—whether it involves challenges, facts, or situations—your neural network will expand. Remember, for this exact reason, variety of diverse experience and travel is critical.

Throughout your lifetime, your neural networks will both reorganize and reinforce themselves according to new mental stimuli and learning experiences. This body-mind/mind-body interaction stimulates our brain cells to grow and connect with each other in complicated ways. This occurs when the branches of nerve fibers (known as dendrites from the Latin word for "tree") expand. Think of dendrites as antennae through which brain neurons communicate with one another. The more dendrites, and the more complex the branches, the better the signal.

Healthy neurons that are well-functioning can be directly linked to thousands of other neurons. This creates a sum of more than a hundred trillion connections, each capable of performing two hundred calculations every second! Basically, the neuron is the structural basis of the brain's thinking ability.

Learning Boosts Brain Power

According to several neuroscientists, the fundamental process of learning and memory comprise transformations between neurons at the synapse level. These changes, termed long-term potentiation (LTP), provide an easy way for neurons to communicate with one another, thus laying the foundation of memory production.

Neuroscientists at Brown University conducted studies that have since provided further evidence that learning uses LTP in order to produce changes in the synaptic connections between brain cells that are needed to gain and store new information.

These researchers conducted studies that taught rats a new motor skill. At the end of the study, scientists discovered that the rats' brains had also changed. They had enlarged, and grown more connections. The more you learn, the better your learning ability becomes. Since you can apply the tips in this book, the mere act of focusing, and learning the tips is actually expanding your brain as you go along.

Cortisol

When your heart is pumping and your body feels ready for action, your brain may be coming under attack by cortisol. This is a hormone you produce when stressed. While stress can temporarily heighten your response, over time, too much cortisol can degenerate the brain and cause more rapid aging. In fact, memory problems and "brain fog" are a common side effect of excess cortisol release. Your brain's hippocampus hates excessive cortisol.

The future in cognitive enhancement and anti-aging will be centered to a great degree around reducing the release of cortisol in the body. Many of the techniques in this book are designed to dramatically reduce cortisol release. Reducing cortisol may help your body cope with stress more intelligently. It also helps to protect you from many degenerative diseases. With the right approach, it is quite easy to control it. For those with fast, pressurized lives, this can really be a lifesaver.

THE THREE KEYS

We're going to look at the three key ways of boosting brainpower. Think of your brain as a super computer. Instead of just looking at intelligence as a single concept, try to see it as the sum of these key components, which combine to produce your thoughts and actions. In order to improve your brain, you need to upgrade and maintain these components regularly:

1. Memory

Your ability to recall information, both in the short term and over many years is vital. Even in our connected age, good memory is a critical component to cognitive processing. Memory is essential to our progress and advancement in life and to our survival.

2. Focus, Concentration & Alertness

In order to harness the maximum potential of your brain, you must be able to focus, concentrate, and, lastly, be alert so that you can take action. By improving these areas, you can make better calculations in life that result in more intelligent decisions and, consequently, better results. This is an essential part of learning how to attain your goals and live a more fulfilling life.

3. Your Processing Speed

A good brain is a quick brain. Being able to make rapid decisions, and to do tasks faster than others, will give you more time and greater output than ever before. Processing speed is the ultimate advantage that you will need in order to succeed. Once you have the information and have retained it, you will need to process that information quickly in order to take action on it. That's where processing speed comes into play.

These three key components act cumulatively. Double your memory capacity, then double your focus and you'll be four times better off. Add some extra processing speed, and you will be well on your way to harnessing the full potential of that not-so-hidden super computer in your head.

FOUR TIER APPROACH

We've found four areas which bring the maximum benefit to your brain with minimum risk.

1. Diet & Nutrition

You are what you eat. Moreover, in many cases, quite literally, your diet is dramatically affecting your brain. The link between nutrition and a healthy and well balanced body is clear. In the same way, what you put into your body will influence what your brain is fed.

2. Exercise

Exercise builds and conditions the brain. We now understand better than ever how exercise affects the brain. We know exactly which physical exercises can actually help make us smarter. The old saying about a healthy mind in a healthy body is spot on. The better your body functions, the better you will be able to think.

3. Supplements

You now have access to what is no less than a box of miracles. There are many naturally occurring and high potency supplements which have been proven to improve your brain in amazing ways. These supplements can give you the extra mental edge that you need. In addition, supplements can help maintain and increase that edge in years to come.

4. Mental Exercise

Like a muscle, the brain grows and develops when trained. New brain training technologies are changing the way we see and exercise our brains. By working your brain, and giving it new tests, you can increase your overall capacity for thought.

1. NUTRITION

Goals:

- Reduce cortisol release.
- Maintain healthy blood sugar.

Cortisol (as discussed earlier) is a stress hormone. Recent studies have shown that it has some of the most negatively impacting effects on cognitive performance. Hypoglycemia or low blood sugar is the second primary culprit which causes impaired brain performance. When it comes to nutrition, we look to these two major areas of focus. In order to succeed in our journey to improve our brain functioning we have to be able to inhibit cortisol release in the body while keeping our blood sugar at a healthy level.

You are what you eat is as true for your brain, as for your body. Optimum nutrition for your mind isn't difficult to grasp, and relies on some simple principles. There is no need to do complex calorie counting, or plan elaborate menus. What you need to focus on is:

- Dramatically reduce carbohydrates.
- Increase protein.
- Eliminate refined carbohydrates.
- Reduce sugar.
- Reduce or eliminate processed foods and foods high in trans fats.

- Eat foods rich in omega three fatty acids.

In addition, adding substances like folic acid, vitamins D and B12, magnesium, and fish oil can aid your thinking processes. Changing your diet for the better, and adding some key supplements may boost your brainpower, and the health of your mind considerably, with little extra effort.

The Energy of Thought and Memory

Did you know that the brain uses over 60% of the body's energy? This is why intense thinking is actually more strenuous than intense physical exercise. The process of thinking is not only tiring, it's exhausting. Needless to say, thinking is a very energy-consuming process. As a result, glucose – the primary source of energy for both the body and the human brain – can be rapidly exhausted during mental activity.

Some interesting research has shown that cognitive abilities actually drain the glucose from a key portion of the brain connected with learning and memory. This emphasizes how crucial glucose is for proper brain performance.

Your brain cells need twice as much energy as the other cells in your body. Neurons, the cells that communicate with each other, have a high demand for energy because they're always in a state of metabolic activity. Even during sleep, neurons are still at work, repairing and rebuilding their worn out or damaged structural components.

Protein

Protein builds up essential neurotransmitters like dopamine, norepinephrine. Protein is essential for proper brain functioning. Dietary protein is our main source of amino acids, the building blocks for both neurotransmitters and body tissues. With the correct balance of amino acids, you can improve your attention span and be able to retain optimum memory and concentration levels for long periods of time.

Protein triggers alertness-inducing neurotransmitters, while carbohydrates trigger drowsiness. Simply put: for maximum brain functioning, you need to eat more protein and less carbohydrates. A good daily guideline is one gram of protein for every two pounds of body weight. If you weigh a hundred and fifty pounds, your daily protein intake should be no less than seventy grams. A can of tuna has twenty-eight grams, and two eggs have sixteen grams. You get the idea. You can get seven grams in a cup of milk or almond milk (unsweetened and fortified with protein powder), or an ounce of cheese or meat. Seek out high protein foods and incorporate them into each meal.

Top Ten Protein Rich Foods

1. Red meat such as beef, pork, and liver
2. White meat such as turkey, chicken and fish
3. Egg whites
4. Dairy products
5. Tuna and other lean fish

6. Legumes and beans
7. Nuts and seeds
8. Algae (Spirulina)
9. Vegetables.
10. Seitan & tofu

Please note: I normally do not recommend either seitan or tofu as they are highly processed but regardless of that fact they are high in protein and low in net carbs. They are often the only real choice for those who don't eat animal products. Seitan is a meat substitute. It is prepared from whole-wheat flour mixed with sufficient amount of water, kneaded and rinsed in water, expelling starch. Finally, although legumes and beans have a high carbohydrate content, this is offset by their high fiber content and minimal effect on the blood sugar. This is known as low NET carbs, which is what we are hoping to accomplish with our diets.

Top 10 Vegetarian Protein Rich Foods

1. Cottage cheese, non-creamed cheese, dry cheese, and non-fat cheese
2. Dried seaweed and spirulina
3. Tofu, seitan or processed meat substitutes
4. Rice protein
5. Pea protein
6. Hemp seeds
7. Nuts such as: cashew nuts, walnuts, and almonds
8. Egg whites
9. Beans

10.   Seeds

Omega 3 Fatty Acids

Omega-3 fatty acids are also known as essential fatty acids. This means that they're essential for human health. Since our bodies cannot produce them, they must be obtained from either food or supplements. Omega-3 fatty acids are found in fish, with the highest levels coming from salmon, blue fin tuna, and halibut. Anchovies and sardines also possess high concentrations of omega-3 fatty acids. Also referred to as polyunsaturated fatty acids (PUFAs), omega-3 fatty acids are vital in both brain function and normal growth and development.

Omega-3 fatty acids are densely concentrated within the brain and appear to be important for both cognitive and behavioral functions. Babies who don't obtain enough omega-3 fatty acids from their mothers during pregnancy risk developing vision and nerve problems. If you're deficient in omega-3 fatty acids, you may experience fatigue, poor memory, mood swings, or depression.

High Protein & Slow Carbs

Health experts have discovered that many people are having success on a so-called "slow-carb diet," which is based on eating foods with a low-glycemic index. Foods with a low GI break down glucose in your body slowly, keeping your blood sugar levels constant throughout the day. No more counting calories on this diet! Just follow the rules and try to keep your meals simple.

Complex carbohydrates release energy gradually and occasionally can be a stable fuel for the body. Simple carbohydrates just pump energy in quickly for a short period, and produce ups and downs which don't help our performance. There is an easy way to tell what you are eating. Complex carbohydrates tend to appear in natural foods, while their simple cousins are usually found in processed junk foods.

When you eat, you are using 20% of your intake for your brain. Eating sugary foods is like dumping a syringe full of energy into the brain, then pulling it back out moments later. On the other hand, eating good, complex carbohydrates gives you a steady supply of energy throughout the day.

Instructions

1. Eat as much as you want of the following foods: proteins (lean meats, poultry, fish, eggs, and cottage cheese); vegetables (except potatoes); legumes (peas, lentils, beans, and nuts); and healthy fats (fish, fish oil, saturated fat, olive oil, and flax seed). Try spreading out your meals, and eating four or five smaller meals a day. This will help balance your blood sugar levels.

2. Avoid eating any white or refined carbohydrates including: white bread, white rice, and white cereals. Even many whole grain breads and cereals are high in carbs and contain high fructose corn syrup. Limit your consumption of those. Look for carbohydrate content and NET carbs. That is the essential factor.

3. Avoid eating fruit daily. Your body converts fruit to fat if you eat too much of it. If you must eat fruits try eating berries or stone fruits as they are some of the lowest NET carb fruits. Avoid eating any kind of junk food or sodas. Stick with water, coffee, tea,

and naturally sweetened drinks with eight grams of carbs or less per serving.

4. Sample meals on this diet might include: eggs (or egg whites) with black beans for breakfast, beef with black beans and mixed veggies, tuna salad with olive oil & nuts, turkey burgers on salad, steak with peas, or grilled chicken and white beans mixed in a green salad. Stock up on canned black beans, white beans, and frozen vegetables, so you will always have them on hand.

When eating out, most restaurants can offer simple solutions to their carb-laden menus. Mediterranean and Mexican restaurants are often happy to replace refined carbs with salad, beans, hummus or veggies. Simply order meals with beef or chicken, and substitute additional black/red beans or vegetables for rice. Beware of added sugar and MSG. These are both brain killers.

Top 10 Brain Foods

There are 47,000 products in the average American grocery store. But, only a handful of these products are great for your brain. Here are my top ten:

1. Whole eggs
2. Lean chicken, beef, lamb, bison or pork
3. Black beans
4. Fish
5. Legumes

6. Lentils

7. Nuts

8. Spinach

9. Broccoli

10. Green beans or peas

10 Foods to Throw Out

Throw those carb rich foods out the window. These starchy items have no place in the diet of a super genius.

1. All bread

2. Rice (including brown)

3. Cereal

4. Potatoes

5. Pasta

6. Tortillas

7. Fried foods

8. Soda

9. Granola

10. Chips

Eating For Intelligence

Breakfast

The old saying that breakfast is the most important meal of the day is no joke. By eating a breakfast containing ample protein and fiber rich "slow" carbohydrates, you will boost your cognitive functioning all day long. Nutritionists at Iowa State University suggest that a breakfast containing ample amounts of protein along with fiber-containing foods is the critical factor in brain nutrition. The combination of fiber and protein helps to keep you satisfied longer, thus stabilizing blood glucose and optimizing your concentration and focus.

Balancing Your Blood Sugar

Whenever you eat foods that contain carbohydrates – excessively sweet or not – your pancreas will secrete a hormone known as insulin. Insulin is vital to our survival, as it pulls excess glucose from foods and stores it for later use. The blood later transfers this excess glucose to other areas of the body that can use it.

Usually, excessively sweet and sugary foods will cause a rapid rise, and equally rapid drop, in blood glucose. As a result, the glucose available for use by your brain has dropped. Your neurons, unable to store glucose, experience a type of energy crisis. Hours later, you feel spaced-out, weak, confused, and/or nervous, dazed or perhaps disoriented. Your ability to focus and think suffers.

This is the hypoglycemia phenomenon we discussed earlier. If allowed to persist it can lead to a lifetime of poor cognitive performance. Think of it this way: If the brain does not have enough fuel to do its work, it will stall. That is exactly what happens when your blood sugar drops.

Eliminating refined carbohydrates, reducing sugar intake to twenty to forty-five grams per day (Yes, this includes fruits and juices and "natural" forms of sugar!) and increasing protein intake can dramatically change the way your brain works. Regulating your blood sugar and blood glucose levels is an essential element in living smarter and longer.

High Sugar Intake over Time

Our bodies and our brains alike are not designed to process refined sugars in the quantities included in modern processed foods. There has been a clear link between excessive sugar intake and diabetes and hypoglycemia. Further complications from sugar-related diseases may cause a narrowing of the arteries. They may make the brain more susceptible to gradual damage. In addition, those with sugar-related illnesses are more vulnerable to depression, panic, and anxiety disorder. They are more likely to suffer a decline in mental ability as they age.

Low Blood Sugar Slows Brain

In order for the brain to function at its full capacity, the body must maintain a steady, healthy supply of blood glucose. If glucose levels drop below a certain level, hypoglycemia occurs. If the level falls too low, disastrous side effects can occur. Dizziness, confusion, impaired judgment, nausea, and appearing intoxicated are common symptoms of hypoglycemia.

In fact, University of Edinburgh researchers concluded that auditory and visual information was processed more slowly when the subjects' brains were temporarily deprived of its main source of energy. That means your intelligence and overall abilities will be severely compromised if your blood sugar levels are not balanced. I can't emphasize enough how critical it is to maintain a healthy blood sugar level. This can be achieved primarily with the diet set forth here, with supplementation, and lastly, with correct exercise.

Glucose, Learning and Memory

Psychology professor, Paul E. Gold, of the University of Illinois College of Medicine is an expert in psychological biochemistry. He has a thing for studying rats. Professor Gold worked with brain expert, Ewan C. McNay. The two were amazed to discover that the brain sometimes can't get enough energy delivered to itself (in the form of glucose) to function properly. It had always been assumed the brain could look after its needs, automatically drawing what it needed.

As they watched rats travel through a maze, they noted that the rats' concentrations of glucose declined in their hippocampus – a key brain region involved in learning and memory. "The new findings suggest that glucose is not always present in sufficient amounts to optimally support learning and memory functions," said Gold.

Just as the body needs calories to function, the brain needs glucose in regulated amounts.

The Glycemic Index

Look for foods with a low GI (Glycemic Index). These foods will keep you stable and focused for longer.

The blood sugar (glucose) that is delivered to the cells throughout our bodies via our bloodstream is partly derived from the carbohydrates in the foods that we eat. A food with a low Glycemic Index (GI) typically only raises blood sugar levels moderately, while a food with a high GI may cause blood sugar levels to spike out of control. When your blood sugar spikes, it is increasing and decreasing rapidly and creating an unstable environment.

Some believe ADHD (Attention Deficit Hyperactivity Disorder) may simply be erratic processing due to a high sensitivity to chemicals in food and the environment, not Ritalin-Deficiency Disease, as some MDs would like to have us think.

Keeping a stable and balanced diet based on GI takes all the guesswork out of eating right. GI values can help us predict the functional effects in our bodies and brains of the carbohydrates we eat. Use the GI as an indispensible tool for helping you select the right foods to help stabilize your blood sugar levels and improve your super genius brain.

2. EXERCISE

Goals:

- Reduce cortisol release.
- Maintain healthy blood sugar.

Most of us know that physical exercise is good for our general health. But, did you know that physical exercise is also good for your brain? If you think you're going to get smarter merely from sitting in front of your computer or watching television, think again. Scientists have discovered that a healthy brain usually lives in an active body.

In order to stay sharp, you must get moving. Exercise can modify proteins that help keep our minds focused, improve memory, and reduce the chance of developing cognitive problems as we age.

The latest in brain science has shown that the key here is short; sharp bursts of exercise on a regular basis. I call this the "resting to rapid" phenomena. These recommendations are made under the assumption that you are in good health, have no pre-existing health conditions and have consulted with a doctor about regular exercise before starting something new and intense. I propose an exercise system that entails taking the heart from resting pace to 90%-97% of your maximum capacity and then holding that for 2-3 minutes. 3-5 sets of that is all you need for optimal brain performance. The theory is very simple: Our ancestors didn't have the luxury of ambling along on a treadmill or steadily swimming laps. They lived active lifestyles which were interspersed with short, life-or-death bursts of action. It is my belief that our bodies function best under these conditions.

You can accomplish all this with just:

- Some form of exercise 4-5 times per week
- Increasing your heart rate for at least 20 minutes per day.

Top Ten "RESTING TO RAPID" Exercises

To get pumped quickly, and release some of those amazing brain chemicals, try these rapid, intense exercises:

1. Jumping rope
2. Biking (stationary or freewheel)
3. Treadmill or outdoor running (maximum speed and incline you can handle)
4. Dance, martial arts or aerobics
5. Rowing machine
6. Fifty-meter sprints
7. Shadow boxing
8. Pushup
9. Swimming
10. Pull ups

Move It or Lose It

Not too long ago, futurists envisioned humans evolving giant thumbs in response to a push-button world. They did not foresee humanity's real response to all its labor-saving conveniences: a sedentary, inactive society with a deteriorated vascular system and consequent decline in physical and mental health.

Unfortunately, almost half of young people from the ages of twelve to twenty-one neglect to participate in any form of vigorous physical exercise on a regular basis. In fact, less than 25% of children report getting at least half an hour of any form of daily exercise. In addition, the same number report that they don't attend their physical education classes in school, either!

In June 2001, ABC News stated that school-aged children spend nearly 4.8 hours per day on the computer, viewing TV, or playing video games. In adults, the problem is even more marked. In fact, the World Health Organization says a sedentary lifestyle is one of the ten leading causes of death and disability. It accounts for 300,000 premature deaths each year in the United States alone. At least half the adults in America don't get enough exercise. A quarter of them get none at all.

This is in sharp contrast from the 1960s, when President John F. Kennedy deemed physical fitness a priority for Americans of all ages.

In our bodies, we have a protein known as brain derived neurotrophic factor, or BDNF. It is produced during exercise. According to MURJ, the undergraduate Research Journal of MIT, BDNF is responsible for creating the synapses between brain cells that move messages. The more synapses we have, the more agile our cognitive activates are in our brains.

In addition, a protein known as beta-amyloid forms plaques in the brain which are purported to progress to Alzheimer's and other dangerous neurological diseases. When animal experiments were conducted using older mice, scientists determined that exercise reduces the amount of beta-amyloid proteins in the brain. Our bodies and our brains are designed to function perfectly when exercised and poorly when we are sedentary. This is a perfect example of literal plaque being built in the brain as a result of not exercising.

Walking

Walking is especially good for your brain. It increases your blood circulation and as well as the oxygen and glucose levels that reach your brain. As you walk, you effectively oxygenate your brain. This is exactly why walking can "clear your head" and help you think better.

Movement and exercise increase both breathing and heart rate. More blood flows to your brain, thus enhancing energy production and waste removal. Studies indicate that, in response to exercise, your cerebral blood vessels can grow.

In one study, senior citizens who walk regularly showed significant improvement in memory skills, compared to sedentary, elderly people.

Not only did walking improve their ability to learn, it improved their concentration and abstract reasoning as well. Stroke risk was reduced by 57% in those who walked for as little as twenty minutes per day.

Running

Neuroscientists at Cambridge University have shown that running stimulates the brain to grow fresh grey matter. Running has a big impact on mental ability.

A few days of running led to the growth of hundreds of thousands of new brain cells that improved the ability to recall memories without confusing them, a skill that is crucial for learning and other cognitive tasks, researchers said.

The new brain cells appeared in a region that is linked to the formation and recollection of memories. This work reveals why jogging and other aerobic exercise can improve memory and learning, and potentially slow down the deterioration of mental ability associated with old age.

Running's brain-boosting effects were in the hippocampus, a region of the brain linked to learning.

Aerobic Exercise

According to the American College of Sports Medicine (ACSM) and other organizations healthy adults under age sixty-four should adhere to the following guidelines for optimal brain health:

Do moderately intense cardio thirty minutes a day, five days a week. This workout can be broken up into sets of three to five minutes at once or throughout the day.

Or

Do vigorously intense cardio twenty minutes a day, three days a week

And

Do eight to ten strength-training exercises, eight to twelve repetitions of each exercise twice a week.

According to the ACSM, "moderate intensity physical activity means working hard enough to raise your heart rate and break a sweat, yet still being able to carry on a conversation. It should be noted that to lose weight or maintain weight loss, 60 to 90 minutes of physical activity may be necessary. The 30-minute recommendation is for the average healthy adult to maintain health and reduce the risk for chronic disease."

Exercise Tips

Everyone is busy, with work, family obligations and/or caring for children. So, it's often hard to get the recommended amount of physical activity. However, the following tips can help pack the most benefit into the tightest routine:

- Exercise in short spurts. Research indicates that exercise of moderate intensity can be met in short three-minute bouts throughout the day. This is great for those of you who are pressed for time. All you have to do is take your heart from resting to 90%-97% of its capacity and repeat as many sets as you can comfortably do.

- Mix it up. You don't need to perform the same routine over and over. Combinations of moderate and vigorous exercise can be used to meet the guidelines. For instance, you can walk briskly for thirty minutes twice per week and run vigorously on one or two other days.

- Set a schedule. Perhaps it's easier for you to exercise during your lunch hour. Or, perhaps hitting the pavement after dinner is best. Regardless of the time, be sure to set aside specific days and times for working out. Make it just as much a regular part of your daily routine as everything else.

In fact, the optimum routine for brain health is easier to plan than you might first think. In order to release the necessary chemicals to reduce cortisol, and improve brain function, you just need to exercise at maximum capacity for short bursts. A "resting to rapid" sprint, and maintaining rapid for three minutes or so is all we need. If we do a set of five sprints at max capacity each day and some strength training twice a week, we can perform at optimal capacity.

You also shouldn't push yourself too hard. Take at least two rest days each week. So, you just need to find fifteen to thirty minutes on five days a week. This is not much to ask for a pumped up brain is it?

- You don't have to go to the gym. Expensive gym memberships aren't prerequisites to getting the required exercise you need. All you need are a pair of athletic shoes and motivation to live a more active and healthy life.

- Exercise with your family. Take your spouse or children along while you exercise. It makes for a nice family outing. In addition, this presents a great role model for encouraging your kids to become more physically active.

- Starting an exercise program to boost your cognitive performance can sound intimidating. However, just remember that your main goal is to boost your brain health by meeting the basic, physical activity recommendations.

- Finally, choose activities that you enjoy, such as: swimming, running, jumping rope, or playing active games with your friends. If you need a variety of exercises to keep you motivated, consider combining a couple of these activities that you enjoy.

3. BRAIN BOOSTERS

Goals:

- Reduce cortisol release.
- Maintain healthy blood sugar.
- Increase memory, focus, and alertness.

Since ancient times, forward thinkers have recognized that, by isolating and extracting specific compounds, powerful mental improvements can be achieved. In order to supercharge your brain, you need added nutrients to take it to the next level. The human body requires at least forty-eight essential nutrients. We will look at those which help the brain and all the ways we can utilize supplements to gain that edge in life.

Boosting your intelligence with supplements is a relatively easy, passive way to see gains. I have very carefully selected the highest performers, and only those supplements which are considered safe to use.

We'll look at the full range of options, including:

- Nootropics/Neuroprotectives to help protect the brain and keep the brain functioning properly.
- Cognitive Enhancers to enhance concentration and memory.
- Adaptogens to help the body adapt to stress.
- Stimulants to aid short-term alertness.

(PS) Phosphatidylserine

Phosphatidylserine (PS) is a fatty acid found in your immune cells and muscle tissue. As well, it is prevalent in your brain cells. PS has many clinically studied benefits for brain improvement, such as enhancing memory, concentration, alertness, and mood. There is some potential for PS to be an active player in cell repair as well. It also helps prevent muscle breakdown due to high cortisol release, and can stimulate your immune response. In some studies, PS has lowered cortisol release by up to 70%!

(Alpha GPC)
L-Alpha Glycerylphosphorylcholine

In the brain, AGPC supports brain function and learning processes by directly increasing the synthesis and secretion of acetylcholine. This is a choline compound that is present within the human brain. It can cross the blood-brain barrier to improve brain functions. Acetylcholine stimulates the cognitive functions that allow a person to focus better. It boosts the Human Growth Hormone (HGH), provides more strength for workouts, and improves the liver's lipotropic functions. Acetylcholine has a positive effect on memory, focus, alertness, clarity and even mood.

VITAMIN B12

Vitamins B12 and B6 help the brain function better. The human brain shrinks with age. This is one major reason why people suffer from Alzheimer's disease. Vitamins B12 and B6 lower the level of homocysteine, an amino acid linked to cardiovascular degeneration. B12 keeps the brain healthy, aids the nervous system, and helps the brain transmit messages.

NIACIN

Niacin is known by a lot of names. It is referred to as vitamin PP, nicotinic acid, and vitamin B3. Niacin supplements have to be taken with food. For best results, you will have to take it with nuts, beans, seeds, and/or yogurt, among other dairy products. Brain researcher, Abram Hoffer, M.D., states that niacin has the ability to cure or reduce: mania, depression, insomnia, and schizophrenia.

DMAE

DMAE or Di-Methyl-Amino-Ethanol can improve your memory and learning abilities. It even boosts intelligence. The human brain already contains some DMAE. However, the level present in a lot of individuals may not be adequate. Several short-term studies have been carried out on DMAE. These studies prove that DMAE can improve alertness, concentration, and focus. DMAE can also lift your mood.

ACETYL L-CARNITINE

ACETYL L-CARNITINE is found in plants. A supplement of this helps people who are suffering from the Alzheimer's disease, and from the aftereffects of stroke. More powerful than normal carnitine, Acetyl-L-Carnitine improves the functioning of human brain. Tests on humans and rats have shown favorable results for treatment of nerve injury in those with Parkinson's disease. Acetyl-L-Carnitine is a non-toxic natural compound.

PEPPERMINT OIL

Peppermint oil soothes the digestive system, provides relief from asthma, and improves cardiovascular health. Its antibacterial properties boost dental health. Research reveals that it improves brain functions, too. Aroma of peppermint oil is believed, by many, to enhance memory, and improve the functioning of the central nervous system. The fact that is opens up the breathing passages which creates an oxygen-rich environment in the brain may add validation to this belief.

HUPERZINE EXTRACT

Huperzine A is present in the Firmoss Huperzia Serrata plant, a rare moss that grows in certain parts of China. Huperzine has been clinically proven to improve memory and learning in animals. Many studies show that it is an invaluable medicine for treating Alzheimer's disease. Huperzine boosts the acetylcholine level within the brain. Acetylcholine is a neurotransmitter that connects the neurons. By improving electrochemical connections, Huperzine treats various diseases, and also enhances memory.

Nootropics / Neuroprotectives

L TYROSINE

L Tyrosine is one of twenty amino acids in the human body. People over forty years might require more supplementation than others. But, we all need it. Trials have shown that L Tyrosine helps the brain respond quickly. It boosts physical as well as cognitive performance. It has shown some effectiveness in treating panic and anxiety disorder, premenstrual syndrome, and depression. More research is currently being conducted. However, the future for L Tyrosine looks promising.

BACOPPA MONNIERI EXTRACT

Bacopa Monnieri is a sacred ayurvedic plant from India. This plant has been used for its medicinal value for thousands of years. It was used to boost intelligence in ancient times. Its antioxidant properties protect mental functions of people with epilepsy. It reduces the effects of stress on the human brain. Extracts of this plant have been shown, in clinical studies, to improve concentration and mental clarity and decrease anxiety, panic and depression. It improves motor learning abilities, according to results of laboratory tests.

VINPOCETINE

Vinpocetine is an extract of the periwinkle plant. It improves brain functions and boosts memory. It provides energy to the brain by delivering glucose and oxygen efficiently. Research has revealed that it improves metabolism in people with tissue damage. It boosts memory and concentration. It can also help in the treatment of Alzheimer's disease and Parkinson's. Vinpocetine can block the dreaded NMDA receptors, which many believe may be responsible for Alzheimer's and other neurodegenerative diseases.

GINKGO BILOBA

Ginkgo Biloba is one of the most studied plants in the world. It is one of the most well-known for its nootropic advantages. Ginkgo Biloba can reduce neurobehavioral dysfunction and brain damage by as much as 50%. According to studies done in France, it may prevent Alzheimer's disease. Scientists at UCLA report that ginkgo biloba may dramatically improve brain functions. It can prevent memory loss and improve attention dramatically in healthy individuals.

CITICOLINE

Citicoline has many names. Some call it INN, while others refer to this as Cytidine 5'-Diphosphocholine or Cytidine Diphosphate-Choline. This unique compound supports the antioxidant defenses of the human body, promotes the neurotransmitter functions, and improves the brain health. Clinical studies have proved that it promotes the ability of a person to learn and memorize. It enhances cognitive functions in conditions such as Parkinson's disease and Alzheimer's.

Adaptogens

Stress is a major factor in all of our lives. It causes physical strain. More importantly, it can wear the mind down. Mental fatigue can impact the body. As a result, we become depleted and exhausted every day. An adaptogen is an herb or nutrient that can improve resistance to trauma, stress, anxiety, and fatigue. Herbalists often refer to adaptogens as rejuvenating herbs. Adaptogens can effectively help balance the human body efficiently and direct it away from stress.

PANAX GINSENG EXTRACT

Ginseng is the root of an herb that has been used in China for centuries. This herb is found in China, Russia, Korea, and in America. It is popular in Greece as "Panax", which means "all heal". Panax Ginseng thus refers to healing all medical conditions. Its main components, ginsenosides, are known for their anticancer, antioxidant, and anti-inflammatory effects. Studies have shown that ginsenosides may treat some cases of diabetes, boost natural immunity, and help in psychological functioning. Panax Ginseng improves brain functions. In China, Panax ginseng is believed to improve memory, concentration, and allow one to clearly focus on a subject. It has worked wonders for people between the ages of thirty-eight and sixty-six. Some traditional Chinese doctors recommend taking it with an extract of the Ginkgo leaf for better results.

RHODIOLA

Depression is a common condition now. Some herbalists believe an extract of Rhodiola Rosea can help. The extract may alleviate depression and lift one's mood. Russian researchers have discovered that rhodiola can increase the resistance to physical, biological and chemical stressors. *The Nordic Journal of Psychiatry* has published these findings. Rhodiola works by changing the levels of dopamine and serotonin. This is useful in both mild and severe depression.

TULSI (HOLY BASIL)

Tulsi, or Holy Basil, is the most sacred plant of ancient India. Ancient Indian Ayurvedic documents list hundreds of medical benefits of this plant. Tulsi is an adaptogen that can balance different physical processes to help a person cope with stress better. Several studies have revealed that this plant can promote longevity, reduce stress, and help create an optimal environment for cognitive enhancement.

Stimulants

A stimulant is anything that stimulates the central nervous system. Often stimulants are seen as productivity enhancers. These enhancers can dramatically affect: alertness, focus, and concentration. For these reasons, stimulants are known to enhance cognitive performance. However stimulants can over-stimulate.

They should be used only in combination with other supplements and in addition to a complete plan as set forth here.

CHOCOLATE

Everybody loves chocolate. Most of us have benefited from its curative abilities too. Chocolate can improve mental function. Its key ingredient is the alkaloid: theobromine. Chocolate can lift one's mood and is known to alleviate depression. Some believe that, particularly in women, chocolate can trigger some of the same emotions as love. Dark chocolates provide the best results because of its higher cocoa content and lower sugar. Ideally eat chocolates where the cocoa content is more than 70%, and avoid more sweetened varieties.

CAFFEINE

Medical evidence proves that caffeine helps people stay alert. Clinical tests have shown that caffeine can enhance performance, improve alertness, and even boost memory. It also improves cognitive performance. For best results however, I recommend green, white, and black tea rather than coffee. Not only does tea contain caffeine but it is also high in a highly-studied alkaloid known as EGCG. EGCG is a powerful anti-oxidant. Besides inhibiting the growth of cancer cells, it kills cancer cells without harming healthy tissue. It has also been effective in lowering LDL cholesterol levels, and inhibiting the abnormal formation of blood clots. EGCG also boasts a host of other neuroprotective and nootropic benefits that may be proven in the future.

KOLA NUT

Kola Nut contains caffeine. This extract is from the Cola Sharp and the Cola Acuminata trees. The nut is smashed to develop a powder or a capsule. It works in the same way as chocolate or caffeine. Take it moderately.

WHITE TEA

Green tea can boost metabolism and help the body in many other ways. Recent research reveals that white tea is also very good. This tea is developed from young buds of the plant. In many Asian cultures, it is believed that white tea can reduce depression and allow for an optimal condition for the brain to relax.

BLACK TEA

In ancient Persia, black tea was used as a medicine for many heart and neurologic conditions. Modern research is now backing up these ancient beliefs in the curative properties of tea. Black tea is believed by most tea drinking cultures to be good for the human brain. This tea has more oxidization, compared to green, white or oolong tea. The flavor is stronger. The caffeine content is also higher in this variety.

GREEN TEA

Far East and Asian people have known for ages about the medicinal properties of green tea. A lot of clinical studies have been conducted in recent times. These tests have shown that green tea contains a compound named polyphenols that can improve the dopamine levels in the brain. Dopamine enhances mood. Some studies show it may even help in hard-to-treat neurological diseases like Parkinson's disease. Another compound phytochemicals provides glucose to the brain. Phytochemicals may prevent heart attacks and cancer. Cultures that drink green tea often have low incidence of cardiovascular and mental illnesses which are high in western cultures. Another active substance in tea known as tannins may boost the brain's functioning as new studies may show.

GUARANA EXTRACT

The guarana plant is found in the Amazon basin. This plant is most famous for its fruit. This supplement is a very powerful stimulant. It has two times more caffeine than you will find in coffee beans yet most people report fewer jitters and more clarity with guarana. Guarana also has a very high nutrient profile. Commonly eaten in Brazil, it is often considered more effective than coffee as a general stimulant.

4. MENTAL EXERCISE

Goals:

- Grow the brain.

- Build neural networks.

When we are young, the world seems filled with curious wonders, delightful discoveries, and daunting challenges. Our brains are taking in countless bits of information and we are developing lifetime skills. This burst of learning is like the brain Olympics of our human journey. Yet, unlike the Olympic athletes who have a limited time to demonstrate their peak performance, the human brain can continue to grow and improve with exercise.

A Simple Brain Exercise

The truth is that, to improve your brain, all you have to do is to carry out things differently. Here is a good brain exercise that can strengthen your neural connections, while creating new ones. It relies on one simple principle: Forcing the brain to do new things is one of the fastest ways to make new neural connections.

First, switch the hand you're using to move the computer mouse. Now, use the hand you normally do not use. What's different? Do you find it harder to be more precise and accurate with your motions? Does it feel as if you're learning to tie your shoes all over again?

If you find this uncomfortable and difficult, don't worry. It's just your brain learning a new skill. This is just like the 'burn' that body builders experience. It means the exercise is working. As you practise more, you'll find this discomfort is reduced as your brain gets stronger. When you feel comfortable, try changing parameters again. Make things tougher.

It's easy to incorporate other neural building exercises with everyday movements. You could use your opposite hand to do common tasks like: brushing your hair; drinking from your water bottle; or changing channels with the TV remote. If you like sports, try using your weaker hand to throw. Or, use the opposite stance when you play tennis or baseball.

Top 10 Brain Exercises

1. Learn a new language.
2. Play chess.
3. Solve Sudoku puzzles.
4. Play video games.
5. Learn to play a musical instrument.
6. Do puzzles.
7. Complete crosswords.

8. Learn a new sport.

9. Read 10% faster than normal.

10. Stop using your calculator or computer to do mathematical calculations. Do them mentally, instead.

Travel

Mental growth comes from new experiences. Exploring new places, stepping out of your comfort zone, and learning about new cultures are all ways to expand your knowledge.

Neurobic Exercises

Neurobics are mental exercises which can enhance and improve the brain's performance. Here are some easy neurobic exercises, which can form a part of your normal day. They all work on the principle of activating normally dormant neural connections, and forcing the brain to build new links and find relationships between new concepts.

Three Keys to Neurobic Exercise:

1. Using multiple senses in combination.

2. Stepping outside your normal comfort zone.

3. Trying exercises which challenge and stimulate your brain.

These keys create a reactivation in the brain. This reactivation causes specific groups of nerve cells to become more active in an unusual pattern. Neurotrophins are a family of proteins that contribute to the development and functioning of neurons. Reactivation in the brain can activate the cells' neurotrophin production and strengthen and build another set of connections in your brain. As the brain develops, you become that much closer to the super genius state.

Sensory Deprivation

For optimum brain function, try to incorporate more of your senses into your daily routine. We usually rely on one major sense for each task. This makes things easier for our brain. To get your mind off the couch and into workout mode, just change things a little with some sensory deprivation.

- Put your clothes on with your eyes closed. Use the sense of touch, and your internal image of your own body, to navigate.

- Share a meal and use only visual cues to communicate. No talking. Or, you might try only using notes. This will make you spell things out clearly.

- Turn the sound off while you watch television. Lip read and guess your way through your favorite program using deduction.

Combine Two of your Senses

Sensory deprivation forces us to think using new inputs. Adding extra stimulation to our brains can also build mental muscle. Instead of focusing on one form of enjoyment, try to build layers of pleasure or activity for your mind.

- Smell roses while you listen to music.
- Listen to the ocean while eating your soup.
- Watch the clouds move, while drawing.
- Get a massage while reading a book.

Change your Routine

Try to look at how your surroundings could be made more interesting for your brain. Just as travel is good for the mind, you can make changes to your routine to give yourself more stimulation.

- Take a different route to work.
- Eat your food with your opposite hand.
- Shop at a different grocery store.

Learning Languages

A great way to change the patterns in our brains is to switch languages. We're so used to hearing English all day that we take in information reflexively, without doing much processing to make sense of it. Make things more of a challenge by introducing some new languages into your life.

- Listen to a foreign language station while working or relaxing.

- Watch the news in another language, or read it online with a translation turned on.

- Buy some audio language programs and learn a few phrases as you drive to work or workout. Watch a foreign film without reading the subtitles.

- Go to a language class once a week, and see if you can hold basic conversation after a month or two.

Imagine Increased Muscle Strength!

For a period of twelve weeks – five minutes a day, five days per week, a group of thirty healthy young adults visualized using either the muscle of their pinky finger or their elbow flexor. Dr. Vinoth Ranganathan and his team at the Cleveland Clinic Foundation asked the participants to imagine they were moving and exercising the muscle that was being tested. He encouraged them to visualize the process in order to make the imaginary movement as real as possible in their minds.

A control group (i.e., those who did no imaginary exercises) showed no strength gains. The little finger group improved their pinky finger strength by 35%. Similarly, the elbow group increased their strength by 13.4%.

This amazing study truly shows how powerful the mind can be. If you can build muscle just by thinking about it, imagine what you could do by building your brain muscle. The possibilities are endless.

Taking Care of Your Brain

Imagine you are training for the Olympics. Yet, every day, you drink, smoke, and eat a double cheeseburger. You'd be building yourself up, and then knocking it all down, never getting anywhere. In the same way, while you train your brain, you should also focus on keeping it healthy and rested. You must literally think about peace of mind.

Socializing

We humans are highly social creatures. As a result, it's hard for us to thrive in isolation. It's even harder for our brains to thrive in isolation. Studies indicate that the more connected we are to other people, the better we perform mentally. Many studies now show that socializing improves our cognitive performance. Our level of social activity can actually prevent diseases like Alzheimer's and boost our daily cognitive performance.

Reducing Stress

We all need to prevent stress from building up. Chronic stress can take a heavy toll on the brain. Stress can lead to shrinkage in the hippocampus region—a key memory area—hindering nerve cell growth, and increasing your risk of developing Alzheimer's disease or dementia. Fortunately, while we can't control the strains of modern life, there are some easy ways to reduce the harmful effects of stress.

Holistic Health

Simple dietary and lifestyle changes are easy to implement. For example, simple supplementation using high quality supplements along with exercise and diet can help to alleviate anxiety and tension, boosting calming chemicals, like dopamine, in the brain. Minimize your intake of high-fat foods, sugar, carbs, and alcohol. Alcohol and refined carbohydrates can elevate stress hormones in our blood, altering our brain chemistry in an unhelpful way.

In addition, MSG*, nitrates, processed foods, strange chemical preservatives, and excess refined carbohydrates can cause anxiety, nervousness, and irritability. Avoiding these foods builds your immunity to stress. A normal, healthy lifestyle is truly the greatest protection.

MSG, a known neurotoxin, is hidden in many foods, particularly processed foods. MSG comes in many different names so do your homework and guard against MSG ingestion.

Hydration

Your body and brain run on food. Both your body and your brain are functioning in an optimal state only if they are also properly hydrated. To improve your brain, you must hydrate!

About 90% of all organic matter is water. The human body is made up of 70% water. Most people are dehydrated and do not drink enough water nor do they take water in the correct way. I suspect many of the medical conditions that drugs are prescribed for often can be attributed to simple dehydration.

Nine Secrets of Hydration

The foundations of most indigenous systems of health and medicine revolve around the basic essentials of life and survival: breathing, drinking, eating, and resting. If balance is achieved in all these areas, your physical health will be in order. A solid system of hydration is no different. It revolves around one thing: balance.

Proper hydration can be one of the critical aspects of maintaining correct balance in health. This system is simple:

1. Drink the correct amount of water for your body weight and level of physical activity. You can find calculators online that will accurately estimate the amount of water you may need based on various factors or, alternatively, use the formula below.

2. Do not over-drink or under-drink. If you over-drink, you eliminate valuable salts and can get bloated. If you under-drink, you dehydrate your body.

3. Sip small amounts of water throughout the day for best absorption. Take three to four sips of water every ten minutes if possible, or five to six swallows every fifteen minutes.

4. Drink the purest and cleanest water you can find. Occasionally, also drink plain unfiltered tap water.

5. If possible incorporate electrolytes and hydration mineral salts into your diet. Effervescent tablets and mineral salts are a great way to accomplish this. Both provide electrolytes that help fluid levels in the body. A bit of sodium boosts absorption. One-third teaspoon of salt per liter of water is about right. There are some amazing sugar-free alternatives out there. Try to find something that is not laden with sugar.

6. Try to drink out of glass whenever possible. Many plastics leach toxins such as the much talked about BPA. Unfortunately, this is unavoidable in our modern world in many cases. Aluminum may be toxic unless it is coated. Metals may leech heavy metal residue. Glass or ceramic is best whenever possible.

7. Start every morning with a four-ounce glass of hot water. This properly prepares the body and digestive track for ingestion.

8. Drink water at room temperature throughout the day and whenever possible. Avoid cold or iced water whenever possible.

9. Limit the amount of other types of beverages until you feel your body is correctly hydrated. Alcohol and caffeine combined dehydrate. Tea is better than coffee. But, until you are properly hydrated, it is better to avoid coffee and alcohol.

How Much Water to Drink?

It's estimated that healthy adults require at least eight to ten cups of water each day. A simple formula is: 0.5 times your weight in pounds to get the number of ounces divided by 8 to get the number of glasses. Example: 115 pounds x .5 = 57.5 ounces; 57.5 divided by 8 equals 7.2 glasses. Drinks such as milk, fruit juices, coffee, tea, and sodas don't count. We need pure clean water whenever possible.

"Thirst kicks in when a person is approximately 1 percent dehydrated," says Ann Grandjean, Ed. D., FACN, executive director of the Center for Human Nutrition in Omaha, Nebraska.

"At two per cent dehydration, thirst becomes more intense, and dry mouth occurs at three per cent." Thirst doesn't always equal dehydration, but it does mean it's time to drink up. If you exercise often and have high levels of physical exertion or live in extreme climates, your needs may be different. Use your intuition and research what the right amounts are for your body type and lifestyle.

Breathe Deep

When you're stressed, your normal breathing rate is altered, sending the oxygen levels in your brain haywire. Decrease your response to problems with deep abdominal breathing. Also known as restorative breathing, this technique is often combined with slow counting. Deep breathing helps you get a physical handle on stress.

A Little Relaxation

It is easy to make excuses for not relaxing. Our modern, busy lives are so hectic that it can feel like an indulgence to relax and take stock. However, making time each day to relax brings big benefits. It will help you perform better at every task, and gives your brain time to grow.

30 SECOND OVERVIEW

Here are the essentials boiled down into a single page. Use this for quick reference.

- Focus your mind on any area of your life which needs improvement.

- Look at the Four Pillars:

    Diet   Neurobics

    Exercise   Supplements

- Use a balanced approach which encompasses brain training, exercise, healthy diet, and good quality supplements.

- Change is the best way to stimulate your brain. Use your senses, routine, location, and sensory inputs to vary your life.

- Look after your brain. Just like athletes must train hard but also take care of their bodies, you need to exercise but be gentle with your mind.

- Never stop learning. You, indeed, can change and grow your brain over your entire life.

FURTHER READING

Though I used many hundreds of sources, including clinical trials, to research this book, for further reading I'd like to recommend some easily digested books which could improve your edge:

1. *Spark: The Revolutionary New Science of Exercise and the Brain* by John J. Ratey and Eric Hagerman.

2. *The 4-Hour Body: An Uncommon Guide to Rapid Fat-Loss, Incredible Sex, and Becoming Superhuman* by Timothy Ferris.

3. *The Brain That Changes Itself: Stories of Personal Triumph from the Frontiers of Brain Science* by Norman Doidge.

4. *Spiritual Intelligence and the Neuroplastic Brain: A Contextual Interpretation of Modern History* by Charles W Mark, PhD.

5. *Train Your Mind, Change Your Brain: How a New Science Reveals Our Extraordinary Potential to Transform Ourselves* by Sharon Begley.

6. *User's Guide to Brain-Boosting Supplements: Learn about the Vitamins and Other Nutrients That Can Boost Your Memory and End Mental Fuzziness* by James J Gormley.

7. *The Health Professional's Guide to Dietary Supplements* by Shawn M. Talbott and Kerry Hughes.

8. *Keep Your Brain Alive: 83 Neurobic Exercises to Help Prevent Memory Loss and Increase Mental Fitness* by Lawrence Katz and Manning Rubin.

9. *Brain Boosters: Food & Drugs that Make You Smarter* by Beverly A. Potter and Sebastian Orfali.

10. *The Man with a Shattered World: The History of a Brain Wound* by Aleksandr Romanovich.

EXCELEROL

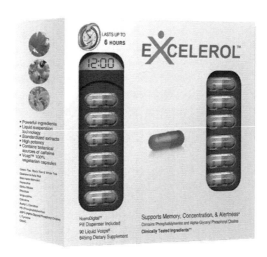

I am sure, by now, after reading about all of the supplements you need to perform at your peak state, you are a little overwhelmed. Taking all those supplements can involve not only a lot of pills but also a lot of money. I know! I used to take over thirty-two pills per day to get my requirements of each of the supplements described here. My monthly supplement bill was over $600 every month. That is why I invented excelerol. I wanted one pill that did it all. After five years of intense product development and research, and in collaboration with one of the largest pharmaceutical companies in the world, I finally released excelerol in the fall of 2011.

There are a lot of great supplements out there. Many are beneficial. But, I truly believe that excelerol represents the cutting edge of supplement technology.

Excelerol is a new nutraceutical dietary supplement. Excelerol supports memory, focus, concentration, and alertness. The ingredients in excelerol are backed by extensive clinical and scientific research.

Excelerol's unique blend of high quality active ingredients and unique liquid capsule suspension technology ensure that you have the highest quality in every capsule. Although many of the ingredients in excelerol, such as citicoline and phosphatidylserine, have a significant amount of scientific-based research, we make no claims as to what benefits you might enjoy from our product.

Excelerol is part herbal supplement and part nutraceutical. Several of its ingredients (like citicoline and phosphatidylserine) may be important chemical nutrients for the brain.

You can learn more about excelerol on the excelerol website:

http://www.excelerol.com

NEURODRIN

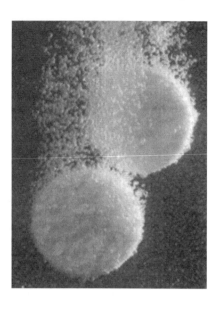

The importance of hydration should not be underestimated in the process of cognitive enhancement. Our second flagship product named neurodrin is a combination of vital nutrients, electrolytes, and many of the plants described here in a flavored, sugar-free, effervescent tablet. This product is awesome when taken in combination with excelerol or as a stand-alone product. Simply add a tablet to your water bottle and enjoy.

ACCELERATED INTELLIGENCE DIGITAL PILL DISPENSER

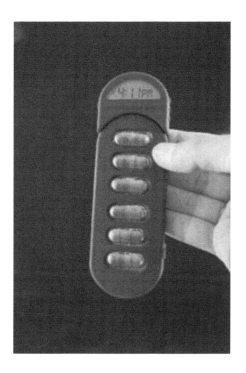

Smart people need a better way to take their pills. The accelerated intelligence (AI) pill dispenser is a unique, pocket-sized device that beeps, illuminates, and vibrates at set intervals to remind you to take your supplements or any other tablets or capsules you need to take for the day.

NEURODRIN INHALER

Recent studies by researchers at the University of Northumbria, Newcastle upon Tyne, in the United Kingdom have discovered that the aroma of peppermint can, in fact, enhance memory. As such, it can be administered by instructors to their students before examinations, to aid in memory, recall and retention. The Neurodrin Inhaler which my company, Accelerated Intelligence Inc., will announce in 2012, will be the first inhaler of its kind anywhere. This unique device will allow a variety of beneficial oils and ingredients, like peppermint, to be inhaled through the nasal passage using a unique patent pending system. An inhalable form of excelerol and neurodrin are also in the works to coincide with the release of this inhaler.

ABOUT THE AUTHOR

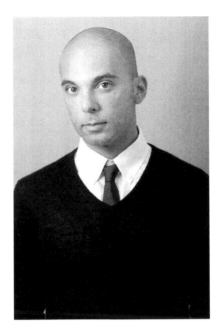

Born in Iran, Shaahin Cheyene is an award winning entrepreneur, researcher, writer, and filmmaker. He is currently based in Los Angeles, California. In the early 1990's, while still in his teens, Cheyene spearheaded the "Smart Drug Movement" by inventing and branding over two hundred award-winning products. Cheyene's products became a global phenomenon, selling millions of units all over the world. Hailed as the "Willy Wonka of Generation X", Cheyene has been compared to such divergent entrepreneurs as Bill Gates and P.T. Barnum. In the early 2000's, Cheyene worked with several major pharmaceutical companies to bring the technologies and benefits of plant medicines to the mainstream. In this process, Cheyene was responsible for the discovery and proliferation of several plant medicines.

In 2000, Cheyene invented, patented, and developed a revolutionary new medicine-delivery technology with the Vapir

Vaporizer, spearheading the then burgeoning vaporization industry. Cheyene is currently the founder of a brain nutrition startup, Accelerated Intelligence Inc., where he is positioning the company to be the leader in the brain nutrition space.

You can learn more about Shaahin Cheyene at www.excelerol.com, or at the author's personal website:

http://www.shaahincheyene.com

Made in the USA
San Bernardino, CA
30 December 2014